Keto Diet for Type 2 Diabetes

How to Manage Type 2 Diabetes Through the Keto Diet Plus Healthy, Delicious, and Easy Recipes!

By: Amy Moore

that the author is not engaging in the rendering of legal, financial, medical or professional advice. The content within this book has been derived from various sources. Please consult a licensed professional before attempting any techniques outlined in this book.

By reading this document, the reader agrees that under no circumstances is the author responsible for any losses, direct or indirect, that are incurred as a result of the use of information contained within this document, including, but not limited to, errors, omissions, or inaccuracies.

Table of Contents

Introduction:Managing Type 2 Diabetes Through the Keto Diet

If you suffer from type 2 diabetes, you already know that managing your diet can be a challenge. The ketogenic diet has become one of the most popular diets in the world now and for good reason. This wonderful diet offers a lot of health benefits – one of which is the improvement of type 2 diabetes.

As a type 2 diabetes sufferer, this is great news for you! This book is all about the ketogenic diet and how you can manage your condition by following it. Congratulations on making one of the best decisions of your life. Your desire to make a healthy change in your life by adopting this diet will allow you to manage your condition more effectively. Through this book, you will discover how easy it is to follow the ketogenic diet and stick with it long-term.

In the first part of this book, we will start off with some background information about type 2 diabetes – what it is, the causes, risk factors, and symptoms of the condition, and how the ketogenic diet can affect it. While you already know that you suffer from type 2 diabetes, this chapter can help you understand your condition better. Having a deeper understanding of your condition, and how the keto diet will affect it, gives you a better idea of how you can follow the ketogenic diet properly to maximize the beneficial results.

After this, you will learn more about the ketogenic diet itself. The ketogenic diet, keto for short, is a low-carb, high-fat diet that includes moderate amounts of protein. While this diet was first developed as part of the treatment for epilepsy, it is now one of the trendiest diets in the world. The second chapter of this book provides you with practical and effective information to help you follow the diet correctly. You will learn what types of foods you can eat, what types of foods you should avoid, and even some practical tips to help you out.

Then, there is a section about cooking on the ketogenic diet. Although cooking on keto doesn't differ that much from cooking on a regular diet, there are some things you have to keep in mind, like the common ingredients and substitutions you can use for keto-friendly dishes, as well as the benefit of learning meal planning. This is an important part of the ketogenic diet as it helps you stick with your diet more consistently by providing you with healthy, tasty options for all your meals throughout the day.

The second part of this book is filled with simple, healthy, delicious recipes that you can whip up in your own kitchen. Whether you decide to start meal planning or not, knowing how to make these dishes will benefit you in different ways. First, we start off with breakfast recipes. All the recipes in this chapter are simple, mouthwatering, and filled with healthy ingredients. Breakfast is the most important part of the day, so if you have the time, you can practice making these dishes to experience first-hand how wonderful it is to follow the keto diet.

Then you will learn several lunch and dinner recipes. The recipes included in this book are so versatile because you can enjoy them at different meals depending on your plan for the day. You can easily interchange the lunch and dinner recipes in this book whether you want to have a hearty lunch and a light dinner or a light lunch and a hearty dinner. Either way, these recipes are so easy that you might even enjoy cooking more and more, which, in turn, helps make the diet easier to follow.

This may come as a surprise to you, but while on keto, you can enjoy desserts – even if you suffer from type 2 diabetes. While the ketogenic diet recommends that you avoid sugar as much as possible, there are many types of sugar-substitutes you can use instead. And these sugar substitutes can easily be used to replace ingredients in traditional dessert recipes, as we have done for you. As with the lunch and dinner recipes, the dessert and snack recipes can be interchanged as well. This means that you can enjoy the desserts as sweet snacks and you can enjoy the snack recipes for dessert after your meals. The dessert and snack recipes included in this book will surely excite you as they are easy to make, delicious, and are only made with keto- and diabetes-friendly ingredients.

While completely reversing type 2 diabetes is rare and difficult, this isn't impossible – especially if you improve your lifestyle and follow the ketogenic diet. This is a concept that is supported by research and medical experts. Throughout this book, you will learn information that will help you manage your condition better. Gone are the days when you have to wonder about what food you should eat, what food you should avoid, and what's the best diet to improve your condition. If you're ready to enrich your life, let's begin!

Chapter 1: Type 2 Diabetes and the Ketogenic Diet

Most diets recommended for people who suffer from type 2 diabetes focus on weight-loss. This is important since most people who have this condition are generally either obese or overweight. Knowing this, you may wonder why the ketogenic diet would be suitable when it focuses on consuming high-fat foods. While it's true that the ketogenic diet is low in carbs and high in fat, it has the potential to change the way your body uses energy and stores fat, thus easing the symptoms of your condition.

Following the ketogenic diet correctly turns your body into a fat-burning machine. This, in turn, may help improve your blood sugar levels, so you don't have to depend too much on insulin. But since this is a special type of diet, it does come with a number of risks. Therefore, it's recommended to speak with your doctor first before you follow the diet. After learning a wealth of useful information from this book, you can have a well-informed conversation with your doctor about the diet and about how you can follow it correctly.

The main goal of the keto diet is to force your body to start burning fat for energy instead of glucose or carbs. While following this unique diet, you would be getting most of your fuel from the high-fat foods you eat while very little of your energy would come from the minimal carbs you consume. While the keto diet recommends high-fat food options, this doesn't mean that you should eat just any types of fats. Following the diet correctly means that you focus on healthy fats from whole, healthy food sources.

Even if you don't follow the ketogenic diet, your doctor may recommend that you limit your carb intake, so you can manage your condition more effectively. This step is crucial since the body converts carbs into sugar, and when you consume large quantities of carbs, this causes spikes in your blood sugar levels – which is never a good thing when you suffer from type 2 diabetes. But when you follow the keto diet, you may experience a reduction in your blood sugar levels.

In the past, one of the most popular low-carb diets recommended for diabetes was the Atkins diet. However, this isn't as effective as keto for managing the condition. The Atkins diet is a high-protein, low-carb diet that has been around since the 1970s. It has often been recommended as an effective way to lose weight and treat a wide range of health conditions, including type 2 diabetes. However, protein can also be converted into glucose by the body. This is what makes the ketogenic diet better – it only recommends the consumption of moderate amounts of protein. That way, your body focuses on burning fat as its main source of fuel.

Straightforward as the ketogenic diet may seem, it does require careful monitoring. An important part of the diet is to count your macros to ensure that you are consuming everything you need to stay healthy and in the appropriate percentages. Then, you should also observe how your body is reacting to the changes in your diet. That way, you can make adjustments to your diet as needed to make sure that you get all the benefits this diet has to offer.

What is Type 2 Diabetes

Diabetes is a type of chronic condition wherein glucose or sugar levels constantly build-up in the blood. Insulin – one of the body's hormones – aids in the transportation of glucose from the bloodstream to the different cells to be utilized for energy. When you suffer from type 2 diabetes, the cells of your body don't respond well to insulin. As the condition becomes more severe, your body starts producing less insulin as well. If left unchecked and untreated, type 2 diabetes may lead to levels of blood glucose that are chronically high, which, in turn, causes adverse symptoms and serious complications.

The good news is that type 2 diabetes can be effectively managed by making some healthy changes to your diet and lifestyle. Doctors can recommend how frequent you must check your levels of blood glucose to ensure that they always stay in a safe range. Apart from the ketogenic diet, here are some other general tips that may help you manage your condition:

- Exercise regularly.
- Eat your meals at regular intervals and avoid skipping meals as much as possible.
- Consume whole, fiber-rich foods to help stabilize your blood glucose levels.

- Avoid overeating. Pay attention to your body so that you can stop eating as soon as you feel full.

Just because you suffer from type 2 diabetes doesn't automatically mean that you would need to take insulin. The only time your doctor would recommend this form of treatment is when your body – specifically your pancreas – isn't able to produce enough of the hormone on its own. If your doctor recommends that you take insulin, make sure you know how to take it properly.

You're lucky if diet and lifestyle changes are enough for you to manage your condition and prevent it from getting worse. But if not, you may have to take some specific medications to help you further manage your condition or help it improve. Some examples of such medications are:

- **Dipeptidyl** to help lower blood glucose levels.
- **Glucagon-like peptide-1 (GLP-1)** to help lower blood glucose levels and slow down the rate of digestion.
- **Meglitinides** to stimulate the pancreas so it releases more insulin.
- **Metformin** to lower blood glucose levels and improve insulin sensitivity.
- **Sodium-glucose cotransporter-2 (SGLT-2)** to prevent the re-absorption of glucose by the kidneys then excreting it in the urine.

- **Sulfonylureas** to help the body produce more insulin.
- **Thiazolidinediones** to increase insulin sensitivity.

As with other types of medications, these may cause a number of potential side effects. Because of this, you may have to try a few medications – and medication combinations – to see which ones are most effective in the treatment of your condition.

In some cases, you may require a treatment known as insulin therapy. Your doctor may recommend this if your body really cannot produce enough insulin. For this treatment option, you may need to take either one injection at night that is long-acting or several insulin doses throughout the day.

While it's not always possible to prevent this condition, there are some ways to delay or slow down its development. To do this, you may need to make some changes to your:

- Diet (try keto – it's really effective!)
- Exercise routine (if you don't have one, start now!)
- Weight management (if you're overweight or obese, try to lose weight!)

The Causes, Risk Factors, and Symptoms of Type 2 Diabetes

Type 2 diabetes is a difficult condition that mainly affects how the body metabolizes glucose or sugar – the body's main fuel source. When you suffer from this condition, two things are happening – either your body cannot produce adequate amounts of insulin or your body resists the effects of this hormone. In the past, type 2 diabetes was referred to as "adult-onset diabetes." However, these days, more and more children are getting diagnosed with the condition, most of whom are either obese or overweight.

Sadly, there is no permanent cure for this condition. But achieving a healthy weight, following the proper diet, and exercising regularly may help you manage type 2 diabetes more effectively. As with other conditions, there are certain symptoms you may manifest if you suffer from type 2 diabetes. If you know that you have a high risk of developing this condition, keep an eye out for the following symptoms:

- Always feeling hungry or thirsty.
- Urinating frequently.
- Sudden and unintentional weight loss.
- Weakness or fatigue.

- Sores and wounds that heal slowly.
- Blurred vision.
- Frequent infections.
- Darkening of the skin in some areas – particularly in the neck and armpits.

If you notice any of these symptoms and you don't see any obvious causes for them, have yourself checked right away for a proper diagnosis. While the exact cause of type 2 diabetes isn't exactly known, there are certain factors that may contribute to its development. The most common risk factors include:

- **Age**

  As you get older, your risk for developing the condition increases, especially when you reach the age of 45 and above. One possible reason for this is that when people reach this age, they tend to gain more weight, exercise less, and lose their muscle mass naturally. However, the occurrence of type 2 diabetes has also been dramatically increasing among young adults, adolescents, and children.

- **Family history**

  If you have a sibling, parent or other close relatives with type 2 diabetes, you may have an increased risk of the disorder too.

- **Fat distribution**

  If you tend to store most of your body fat in your abdomen, this increases your risk of the condition compared to when you store your body fat in your thighs, hips or any other part of your body.

- **Gestational diabetes**

  When pregnant women develop this condition during their pregnancy, this increases their risk of developing type 2 diabetes as well. The same thing goes for when a woman gives birth to an infant who weighs over 9 pounds.

- **Inactive or sedentary lifestyle**

  The more sedentary your lifestyle is, the more at-risk you are for developing this condition. Remaining physically active helps you maintain a healthy weight as it helps you use your energy, thus improving your insulin sensitivity.

- **Obesity**

  This is one of the main risk factors for the condition. Of course, you don't always have to be obese or overweight to experience type 2 diabetes.

- **Polycystic ovarian syndrome (PCOS)**

This is a condition that's commonly characterized by excess growth of hair, obesity, and irregular menstrual periods. Having this condition is also a risk factor for type 2 diabetes.

- **Prediabetes**

  This is a related condition wherein your levels of blood sugar are higher than normal but not enough to be diagnosed with diabetes. If left unchecked and untreated, this condition may progress to type 2 diabetes.

- **Race**

  Health experts don't really know why people of certain races are more susceptible to this condition. Such races include Asian-American, African-American, American Indian, and Hispanic.

It's important to seek immediate treatment when you know that you already suffer from this condition. Otherwise, you might experience the many complications that can potentially occur when the condition is left untreated. Some of the more common complications of type 2 diabetes are:

- Alzheimer's disease.
- Blood vessel and heart disease.
- Eye damage.

- Hearing impairment.
- Kidney damage.
- Nerve damage, particularly the nerves responsible for digestion.
- Neuropathy or nerve damage.
- Skin infections and other issues.
- Sleep apnea.
- Very slow healing of blisters, cuts, wounds, and sores.

How Does the Ketogenic Diet Affect Type 2 Diabetes?

Now that you have a better understanding of type 2 diabetes, it's time to learn how the ketogenic diet can affect the condition. As previously mentioned, managing this condition is possible by making some changes to your diet and lifestyle. When it comes to your diet, one of the most significant things you can do to improve your type 2 diabetes is to follow the ketogenic diet – a unique type of diet that is high in fat, low in carbs, and allows for moderate protein intake.

Research and anecdotal evidence suggests that this diet can be highly beneficial for anyone who suffers from type 2 diabetes. Foods that are high in carbs such as milk, rice, starchy fruits, bread, and pasta are very common in traditional diets. When you follow a diet wherein you eat a lot of these types of foods, your body makes use of insulin to transport glucose from these foods from your bloodstream to the different cells of your body to be used for energy.

Unfortunately, because of your condition, your body either cannot produce adequate amounts of insulin or your body doesn't use insulin properly. Either condition affects how your body utilizes carbs, which, in turn, causes you to experience frequent spikes in your blood sugar levels. This means that whenever you consume meals that are high in carbs, you can expect your blood glucose levels to go through the roof!

The good news is that the main concept of the ketogenic diet is to limit your intake of foods that are high in carbs and sugar. Because of this, following the diet may:

- Reduce your risk of developing both type 1 and type 2 diabetes – if you don't suffer from it yet.
- Improve your body's glycemic control if you already suffer from the condition.
- Help you lose weight, which comes with a lot of other health benefits.

Making a choice to follow the keto diet means that you are also making a choice to give up your carb-rich eating habits. After some time – when you have successfully "starved" your body of carbs – your body is forced to break down the fatty foods you eat and even your body's fat stores for fuel. This is a natural metabolic process that results from the ketogenic diet, and it is known as ketosis. When you achieve a state of ketosis, your body starts producing ketone bodies or "ketones" for fuel.

In the long-term, this diet may help you control your blood sugar levels more effectively. This diet is beneficial for type 2 diabetes because it helps lower these levels and maintains them at healthy levels. Also, the restriction of carbs helps eliminate the occurrence of large and frequent spikes in your blood sugar, thus reducing your need for insulin.

As your blood sugar levels go down, your doctor may reduce the number of medications you need to take. This is one of the most important benefits of the diet because a lot of the medications taken for this condition may have potential side effects. But you should never decide to reduce or stop taking your diabetes medications on your own. Your doctor is the one who should make this decision based on how your body benefits from the diet and how much of an improvement you have experienced because of it.

It's also important to note that if you are undergoing insulin therapy, going keto might not be the best option for you as it might increase your risk of developing a condition known as hypoglycemia. The same applies to when you are taking different types of medications. In such cases, speak with your doctor first before starting the ketogenic diet. That way, you can combine the knowledge you have learned through this book with the information your doctor will share with you. Together, you can even come up with a specialized keto diet plan to improve your condition.

Since the ketogenic diet basically turns your body into an efficient fat-burning machine, weight-loss is one of the most common benefits of this diet too. If you are obese or overweight and this has made your condition worse – or even contributed to its development – you'll be happy to know that you can potentially lose a significant amount of weight through this diet. This is especially true if you follow it correctly. When you lose weight, this may also improve your glycemic control, energy distribution, and overall well-being.

Chapter 2: Following the Ketogenic Diet

If you are interested in following the ketogenic diet for the benefit of your condition, then you should learn all the basics of going keto. Educating yourself is an important step because it will allow you to follow the diet correctly – this is crucial if you want to maximize all the good benefits this diet has to offer. This low-carb, high-fat diet has become widely popular in the past few years because of its health benefits such as weight loss, overall health improvement, and more. But when starting the diet, you may feel quite overwhelmed – especially if you are used to a high-carb diet that includes a lot of processed, packaged, and ready-made foods.

In order to successfully start the diet – and stick with it long-term – you must know the types of foods to eat and avoid. This information is the foundation of the ketogenic diet and knowing it is essential. Fortunately, you will learn all this basic information in this chapter! Here, you will find out exactly what kinds of food you can eat, what kinds of food you should eliminate or restrict from your diet, and even some practical keto diet tips to help you out. This information will give you a clearer picture of what the diet really looks like.

Foods to Eat on the Ketogenic Diet

Basically, the keto diet recommends you to eat high-fat foods, minimal carbs, and moderate amounts of protein. If this is the first time you have ever tried following a diet before, then restricting your carb intake might be the most challenging thing to do – challenging, but not impossible. Here's more good news for you, the longer you stick with the ketogenic diet, the less you will crave the foods you must avoid.

Generally, when you follow the ketogenic diet, 75% of your daily calories should come from fat, 20% from protein, and only 5% from carbs. This means that you would only be eating about 30 grams of carbs a day. It's important to follow these macros percentages consistently each day if you want to reach and maintain ketosis. It's never a good idea to follow the diet one day then consume a lot of carbs the next. This will not only confuse your body, but it will also cause spikes in your blood sugar levels. To give you a better idea of what foods to eat on keto, here is a general list for you:

1. Berries

When it comes to the ketogenic diet, most types of fruits aren't recommended, mainly because they contain a lot of carbs and sugar. However, berries are the exception to the rule. Although berries have a pleasantly sweet taste, they are low in carbs but high in antioxidants and fiber. You may enjoy a handful of berries as a snack or even include them in your recipes. Some examples of berries are:

- Blueberries
- Cherries
- Cranberries
- Mulberries
- Raspberries
- Strawberries

2. Collagen

If you need an extra boost of protein, you can get it from collagen, preferably the grass-fed variety. This usually comes in powder form and you can mix it into any recipe or drink to add protein without changing the taste.

3. Dairy

Since dairy products are high in fat, they are recommended on the keto diet – just make sure that you know the exact carb content of the dairy products you consume at each meal. Cheese is one type of dairy that is high in fat. Most types of cheese contain more than 30% fat, making it great for keto. Cheese also contains good amounts of protein and calcium, both of which are essential. One issue you may have to look out for when it comes to cheese is portion size.

Counting macros is important on keto, and you should know that there are some types of cheese that may contain up to 30% of your RDA for saturated fat. So if you do include cheese in your diet, limit your portions. When it comes to cheese, the best types for keto are hard cheeses such as feta, cheddar, parmesan, or Swiss, and soft cheeses like blue cheese, Monterey Jack, brie, or mozzarella.

Another great dairy option for keto is plain Greek yogurt as it contains good amounts of calcium and protein. Make sure to stick with the plain variety because flavored yogurt products are typically high in sugar. Aside from being suitable for the keto diet, Greek yogurt also supports weight loss by helping to reduce your appetite. Other dairy products you may have include:

- o Full-fat yogurt
- o Heavy cream
- o Mayonnaise
- o Sour cream

○

4. Dark Chocolate and cocoa powder

When searching for dark chocolate to eat or to include in your recipes, opt for those which contain a minimum of 70% cocoa solids – the darker, the better. Dark chocolate and cocoa powder contain antioxidants that provide a number of health benefits to support your overall health.

5. Eggs

These are great too because you can eat them in a variety of ways. Eggs are tasty, extremely versatile, high in protein, and contain almost no carbs. Another nutrient you may get from eggs is vitamin D, which is an essential fat-soluble vitamin.

6. Fats and Oils

Try to incorporate a lot of fats and oils into each meal you eat, especially when you are having a particularly low-fat meal like a light salad. Adding healthy fats and oils to your meals makes them taste better and makes them more suitable for your diet as well. Some healthy fats and healthy fat sources to use include:

- Avocado
- Butter
- Coconut oil
- Duck fat
- Ghee
- Lard
- Macadamia nuts
- Olive oil

7. **Fish and Seafood**

Fatty fish like tuna and salmon are the best options, especially when roasted, grilled, or sautéed. Try to avoid breading fish and seafood as this adds carbs to the dish. Fish and seafood are great protein sources and most options are free of carbs. Some examples of this food group are:

- Catfish
- Clams
- Cod
- Crab
- Halibut
- Mackerel
- Mahi-mahi
- Mussels
- Octopus
- Oysters
- Lobster

- Shrimp
- Squid

8. **Non-Starchy Vegetables**

Most low-carb vegetables are the ones that grow above the ground – either frozen or fresh. Green, leafy veggies are rich in nutrients and tossing them in butter, oil or other kinds of high-fat dressing is an excellent way to add healthy fats to your diet without adding too many calories. Vegetables are also important because they are high in antioxidants. These help combat oxidative stress while eliminating toxins from the body.

Also, most dietary guidelines recommend the consumption of a minimum of five cups of vegetables and fruits each day. Since most fruits aren't recommended on keto (although you may still enjoy them once in a while – just make sure that they don't cause you to go over your daily carb requirement), you should try to increase your vegetable intake. Some of the best vegetables to include in your diet are:

- Asparagus
- Bok choy
- Broccoli
- Cabbage
- Cauliflower
- Celery

- Chives
- Cucumber
- Endives
- Kale
- Lettuce
- Radicchio
- Radishes
- Spinach
- Swiss chard

Although chili and bell peppers are technically fruits, these are recommended for the keto diet as well. This is because they contain specific compounds that increase metabolism and promote ketosis, so you can burn more calories each day.

9. Nuts and Seeds

Although nuts and seeds contain carbs, they also contain high amounts of healthy fats, and they're healthy for the heart too. However, as with dairy, it's best to control your portion size for this food group. As a snack, you should only consume a handful of nuts or seeds. The same thing goes for using them in recipes – don't use too many as this may drive up the carb and overall caloric content of your dishes. Some great options for nuts and seeds include:

- ○ Almonds
- ○ Brazil nuts
- ○ Chia seeds
- ○ Hazelnuts
- ○ Macadamia nuts
- ○ Peanuts
- ○ Pecans
- ○ Pine nuts
- ○ Walnuts

10. Protein

When it comes to protein, try not to go overboard as consuming excessive amounts of protein may increase your glucose levels too. When this happens, your body cannot go into ketosis. Make sure to choose fresh meat to get high-quality protein for your diet. Also, meat provides you with zinc, potassium, and other essential minerals needed to stay healthy. B vitamins are another important component of meat as they help with the body's process of extracting energy from the foods you eat. Some great sources of protein to enjoy on the keto diet are:

- ○ Bacon (yes, bacon!)
- ○ Beef
- ○ Goat
- ○ Lamb
- ○ Organs

- Pork
- Poultry

Also, when it comes to meat, opt for pasture-raised and grass-fed varieties as much as possible.

Foods to Avoid on the Ketogenic Diet

If there are foods that you should eat while on keto, there are also foods you must avoid. Knowing these foods will help you plan your meals better, thus making it easier for you to stick with your diet. While on keto, avoid the following.

1. **Alcohol**

   While not all types of alcoholic beverages must be avoided on this diet, it's recommended to limit your alcohol consumption, especially at the start of the diet and if you want to lose weight faster. Hard liquors are okay, but when it comes to these beverages, stay away from beer, cocktails, and other alcoholic concoctions that contain sweet ingredients.

2. **Beans and Legumes**

   Most beans and legumes are high in starch, thus making them a no-no for keto. Also, these foods are relatively low in fat, which means that they won't contribute to your daily fat intake. Some examples of beans and legumes to avoid are:

- ○ Black beans
- ○ Chickpeas
- ○ Kidney beans
- ○ Lentils

3. Grains

All types of grains and foods that contain grains must be avoided in order to successfully follow the diet. The fact is, grains are high in carbs, so when you continue eating them, there's a very slim chance that you will reach ketosis. Some examples of grains to avoid are:

- ○ Barley
- ○ Bread
- ○ Buckwheat
- ○ Cakes
- ○ Cereal
- ○ Pasta
- ○ Pastries
- ○ Quinoa
- ○ Rice
- ○ Wheat
- ○ Whole grains

4. Starchy Fruits and Vegetables

Apart from berries, you should limit your consumption of fruits – including fresh fruit juices and smoothies. In particular, large fruits are very high in sugar. Starchy vegetables – most of those that grow underground – are high in carbs and calories too. Here are some types of starchy fruits and vegetables to stay away from:

- ○ Apples
- ○ Bananas
- ○ Corn
- ○ Grapes
- ○ Mangoes
- ○ Oranges
- ○ Papayas
- ○ Pineapples
- ○ Potatoes and potato products
- ○ Sweet potatoes
- ○ Tangerines
- ○ Yams

5. Refined or Trans Fats and Oils

While fats and oils are recommended for the keto diet, not all of these are healthy. While on keto, make sure to focus on healthy fats instead of the following:

- ○ Canola oil
- ○ Corn oil
- ○ Cottonseed oil
- ○ Grapeseed oil
- ○ Margarine
- ○ Safflower oil

- Soybean oil
- Spreadable butter alternatives
- Sunflower oil

6. Sugar

While avoiding sugar as part of the keto diet is beneficial for most people, it is especially beneficial when you suffer from type 2 diabetes. Consuming a lot of sugar and sugary foods leads to weight gain along with an increased risk of developing various chronic illnesses. When it comes to sugar, here are some examples of foods to avoid:

- Agave
- Breakfast cereal
- Cakes
- Candy
- Chocolate
- Honey
- Juice
- Maple syrup
- Soda
- Sports drinks

Tips for Following the Ketogenic Diet with Type 2 Diabetes

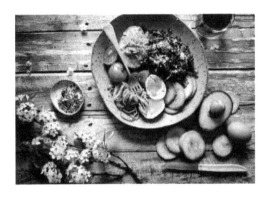

Different as the ketogenic diet may be from your current diet, following it doesn't have to be difficult. Since you will be avoiding foods that cause your blood sugar levels to spike, you may start seeing improvements in your condition after some time, as long as you follow the diet correctly. To do this, here are some tips to guide you:

1. **Personalize your intake of carbs based on your own needs**

   While the ketogenic diet recommends that you avoid carbs, there are different types of ketogenic diets you can follow, and they allow for varying macros breakdowns. If this is your first time to start keto, you should gradually reduce your carb intake instead of quitting cold turkey. Plan your carb intake reduction to ensure that your body doesn't get shocked and you don't feel too challenged. Even though you have to limit your carb intake, it may require some experimentation for you to find the best percentage of carbs to make you feel healthy and happy while still being able to achieve ketosis.

2. **Focus on healthy fat and protein sources**

   When planning your meals and shopping for ingredients for your recipes, opt for healthy, whole food sources instead of the processed varieties. For instance, fresh meat, eggs, dairy, and fish would make you a lot healthier than only eating cured, processed or packaged food items. Also, when choosing oils, opt for the ones that contain poly- and mono-unsaturated fats instead of saturated or trans fats.

3. Eat a lot of fiber-rich foods too

If you have to eat foods that contain carbs, try to choose those which also contain a lot of fiber. Apart from making you feel full for a longer time, fiber also helps lower your levels of LDL cholesterol.

4. Choose sugar substitutes and sweeteners wisely

While following the keto diet, you can still enjoy sweet foods – the only difference is that they would be made with healthier sugar substitutes and sweeteners. When choosing such flavor enhancers, choose wisely. Some sweeteners, although they won't impact your blood sugar levels, might increase your craving for sweet and sugary foods. Also, avoid sugary food items that contain sugar alcohols as some of these may affect your blood sugar levels. Because of these dangers, it's recommended to make your own sweet desserts and snacks so that you can choose what goes into them to ensure that you only eat keto- and diabetes-friendly sweet treats.

5. Know which foods are low on the glycemic index

Counting your macros is important on the keto diet. Another way you can keep track of the foods you eat is by using the glycemic index. This provides you with a better idea of how your body may respond to certain foods when you suffer from type 2 diabetes. Use it as a supplementary tool only because it doesn't provide information about the complete nutritional values of foods.

With all the health benefits of the keto diet, you might wonder if it can reverse your condition.

In some cases, yes, it can.

Advocates of this diet claim that it helps restore insulin sensitivity, which, in turn, causes the symptoms of diabetes to go away. When you follow this diet correctly – and you work hand-in-hand with your doctor throughout the process – you may be able to manage your condition well. After some time, your doctor might even cease your insulin medications entirely.

The reversal of type 2 diabetes is one of the best benefits you can get from the ketogenic diet. Of course, reversal, in this case, doesn't always mean permanence. Once you stop following the diet, the symptoms of your condition might return after some time. Therefore, if you choose to go keto, you may have to set your mind to follow it long-term. If it works for you, stick with it for the improvement of your overall health.

Speak to Your Doctor First!

This is another important tip that has been repeated in the previous chapters because of how important it is. Even when you are at the peak of health, it's recommended to speak with your doctor before starting any new diet or eating plan – including keto. Since you suffer from type 2 diabetes, a condition that requires constant monitoring, consulting with your doctor is even more important. If you suffer from this condition, your doctor can help you with:

- Learning how to monitor your levels of blood glucose at home.
- Dietary recommendations, including a customized keto diet plan to suit your own individual needs.
- Recommendations for exercises and physical activity you can do while on keto.
- Information regarding medications that you need to take – or discontinue – while following the ketogenic diet.

It's also important for you to keep visiting your doctor – especially at the beginning – in order to observe and monitor the progress of your condition. Over time, when your body has adjusted to your diet, you can reduce the frequency of your consultations. But if you experience any new symptoms – especially adverse symptoms – consult with your doctor right away.

Chapter 3: Cooking on Keto

When you suffer from type 2 diabetes, it's like your body is suffering from carbohydrate intoxication. When you have been consuming carbs in high amounts, this eventually causes your body to be overwhelmed with carbs – so much that you develop insulin resistance. It's like your cells are saying, "enough with the carbs and sugar!" so you develop a condition that forces you to become more aware of your body.

As you transition to the ketogenic diet, which is high in fats and low in carbs, you may start seeing improvements in your condition. When you are able to achieve ketosis, your body won't need a lot of insulin, and this gives your body the opportunity to correct itself. If you are in the early stages of type 2 diabetes, you may want to speak to your doctor about going keto first before you start taking insulin or other types of medications. With this new diet – and other healthy changes to your lifestyle – you may be able to improve your symptoms even before your condition worsens.

As long as you have committed yourself to follow the ketogenic diet – and you really follow it correctly – you may start experiencing small improvements in the levels of your blood sugar in a matter of days. After a few weeks, you may be able to notice – and feel – a significant shift in these levels.

If you're ready to start following the ketogenic diet, you should know that cooking is a significant part of it. Learning how to cook for your keto diet keeps you motivated and allows you to stick with the diet long-term. Before we move on to some simple but healthy recipes to incorporate into your meal planning, let's discuss the common ingredients to use for keto-friendly dishes along with meal planning – another important part of the keto diet you may want to consider.

Basic Ingredients for Cooking on Keto

Don't allow yourself to get overwhelmed or intimidated as you start cooking on keto. If you have been cooking for yourself in the past, cooking on keto would be a breeze for you. But even if this is your first time to cook, starting with simple recipes will give you the confidence to keep cooking and keep following your new diet.

Cooking your own meals is one of the best ways to motivate yourself and make you feel happier about the life-changing decision you have made. Learning how to cook on keto is an important skill to build your foundation of healthy breakfast, lunch, dinner, dessert, and snack recipes to make each day.

As with any other diet, going keto requires dedication, discipline, and a drive to follow the very specific requirements of the diet – eating high-fat, moderate-protein, and low-carb foods. While there are different types of ketogenic diets, most beginners start with the Standard Ketogenic Diet (SKD). This variation recommends 70 to 80% fat, 10 to 20% protein, and 5 to 10% carbs. If you want to lose weight on this diet too, you may need to consume less than 2,000 calories each day – then plan your meals to meet the proper percentages of the SKD.

After choosing the type of keto diet to follow, it's time to start planning your meals. But before you can do that, you may want to familiarize yourself with the basic ingredients used for keto cooking. Of course, the shopping list you make would depend on the meals you have planned to cook for the week. To give you a better idea of basic cooking ingredients you may use on keto, here are some common examples:

Fresh produce

- avocado
- cabbage
- cherry tomatoes
- garlic
- leaf or romaine lettuce
- lime
- mushrooms
- onions
- red bell pepper
- scallions
- spinach

Oils and spices

- avocado oil
- butter
- cinnamon
- coconut oil
- garlic powder
- ground ginger
- salt
- pepper
- sesame oil
- sesame seeds

Protein sources

- bacon
- breakfast sausages
- chicken breasts (boneless, skinless)
- cream cheese
- eggs
- dairy
- ground beef
- mozzarella cheese
- plain yogurt

Staple pantry ingredients

- almond butter
- almond flour
- chicken broth
- cocoa powder
- coconut cream
- soy sauce
- vanilla extract

Meal Planning

As a sufferer of type 2 diabetes, following the ketogenic diet is one of the best things you can do for your health. You won't have to deprive yourself while on this diet – you just have to make smarter choices. And one of the most effective ways to stick with your diet is to start meal planning.

Meal planning is a process that involves planning your meals (usually for a week), coming up with a list of ingredients, shopping for those ingredients, preparing and cooking your meals, and storing them in the refrigerator to keep them fresh. Meal planning saves time, money, and keeps you more motivated to stick with your diet long-term. The key to meal planning is to build your own file of recipes that you like and that are suitable for your new diet. When meal planning, here are some tips to keep in mind:

- Start off with easy and simple recipes that will help you practice basic cooking skills, thus preparing you to make more complex recipes in the future.
- When looking for recipes, opt for those that offer versatility in terms of what ingredients you can use for them.
- Make sure that all the meals you have planned allow you to complete your required macronutrient profile for the day.
- Also, make sure that the meals you have planned don't go beyond the caloric requirement for the day.

-
- Opt for low-carb, high-fat, and moderate-protein recipes and when planning, combine them in such a way that you get high amounts of fat, moderate amounts of protein, and low amounts of carbs each day.
- Opt for more seafood and fish recipes for healthier protein sources.
- When it comes to choosing dairy products for your recipes, opt for whole-fat.
- If your planned meals don't have enough calories, pair it with low-carb side dishes that feature non-starchy vegetables.

Chapter 4: Keto Breakfast Recipes for Type 2 Diabetes

Now that you have a better understanding of the keto diet and how it relates to and benefits type 2 diabetes, let's take a look at some easy, tasty, and healthy recipes. Since breakfast is the most important part of the day, let's begin with some breakfast recipes. When it comes to choosing breakfast dishes, make sure that this meal contains all the healthy nutrients you need to start your day right. That way, you will have all the energy you need to get through the morning without getting hungry until it's time for lunch.

Turkey Bacon Egg Muffins

These healthy muffins are made with eggs, turkey bacon, and other healthy ingredients. Making them is a breeze and it doesn't take a lot of time either. If you want a quick breakfast that tastes great and stores well (for meal planning), then this

is the perfect recipe for you to start with.

Time: 35 minutes

Serving Size: 12 egg muffins

Ingredients:

- 1 tsp pepper
- 1-½ tsp salt
- ¼ cup spinach (chopped)
- ⅓ cup bell pepper (chopped)
- ⅓ cup turkey sausage (lean, chopped)
- ⅓ cup yellow onion (chopped)
- ½ jalapeño pepper
- 1 garlic clove
- 3 small eggs
- 12 medium eggs (whites only)
- 12 slices of turkey bacon (lean)

Directions:

1. Preheat your oven to 350°F and grease a muffin pan.
2. Surround each of the muffin cups with a slice of turkey bacon.
3. Place some chopped spinach at the bottom of each muffin cup.
4. In a pan, sauté the garlic, onions, and jalapeño until the onions have turned translucent.
5. Take the pan out of the heat and spoon the cooked vegetables on top of the spinach.
6. Top with the chopped bell pepper and sausage.
7. In a bowl, combine the small eggs and egg whites, then season with salt and pepper. Whisk together well.
8. Spoon the egg mixture into the muffin cups until you have covered the other ingredients completely.
9. Place the muffin pan in the oven and bake the egg muffins for about 25 minutes.
10. Take the muffin pan out of the oven and allow the muffins to cool before serving or storing.

Cinnamon Orange Muffins

Enjoy these cinnamon orange muffins during the holidays or at any time of the year. These low-carb muffins have a unique flavor that you will surely crave for over and over again. They're easy to bake and they go perfectly well with tea or coffee.

Time: 30 minutes

Serving Size: 12 muffins

Ingredients:

- ¼ tsp cloves
- 1 tsp baking soda
- 1 tsp lemon juice
- 1 tsp nutmeg
- 3 tbsp cinnamon
- 3 tbsp orange zest
- ½ cup ghee (melted)
- 3 cups almond flour
- 4 large eggs (whisked)
- keto-friendly sweetener

Directions:

1. Preheat your oven to 350°F and grease a muffin pan.
2. In a bowl, combine all the measured ingredients and add sweetener to taste. Mix well until all ingredients are well-incorporated.
3. Pour the batter into the muffin pan.
4. Place the muffin pan in the oven and bake the muffins for about 18 to 20 minutes.
5. Take the muffin pan out of the oven and allow the muffins to cool down.

Cheesy Mushroom and Spinach Quiche

This low-carb quiche will tickle your taste buds and satisfy your breakfast cravings. It's easy to make and it would take you less than an hour. You can make the quiche with a crust or without it – either way works! For this recipe, you will be making a crustless quiche – perfect for keto!

Time: 45 minutes

Serving Size: 1 quiche

Ingredients:

- ½ tsp garlic powder
- ⅓ cup parmesan cheese (shredded)
- ½ cup heavy cream
- ½ cup of water
- 1 cup mozzarella (shredded)
- 1 cup mushrooms (sliced)
- 1-¼ cups spinach
- 2 slices of provolone cheese (or any other kind of cheese)
- 6 large eggs
- black pepper
- salt

Directions:

1. Grease a pie pan and spread the spinach leaves on the bottom.
2. Top evenly with a layer of mushrooms, then with the cheese slices, and set aside.
3. In a bowl, combine the water and heavy cream and whisk well.
4. Add the garlic powder, parmesan cheese, and a pinch of salt and pepper then continue mixing.
5. Pour the mixture over the spinach and mushrooms.
6. Sprinkle generously with mozzarella.
7. Place the pie pan in the oven and bake the quiche at 350°F for about 40 minutes.
8. Take the pie pan out of the oven and allow the quiche to cool before slicing.

No-Bread Breakfast Sandwich

This is an inventive sandwich that was made for keto since it has no bread! The sizzling ham, scrumptious cheese, and healthy eggs come together in perfect combination for this one-of-a-kind keto sandwich. It's easy, delicious, and quick to make too.

Time: 10 minutes

Serving Size: 2 sandwiches

Ingredients:

- 2 tbsp butter
- ¼ cup cheddar cheese (sliced thickly)
- 2 slices of deli ham (smoked)
- 4 medium eggs
- black pepper
- salt
- Tabasco sauce (optional)

Directions:

1. In a pan, add the butter over medium heat.
2. Add the eggs and fry over easy. Season with salt and pepper.

3. Assemble your sandwich. Start with the eggs as the base, place a slice of ham then top with cheese slices. Top off each sandwich with another fried egg.
4. Turn the heat down to low and place the sandwiches back on the pan.
5. Continue frying until the cheese melts then transfer to serving plates. Add a few drops of Tabasco sauce if desired.

Smoked Salmon Wraps with Cream Cheese

Simple as this breakfast recipe is, the combination of cream cheese and salmon happens to be the most iconic combination for breakfast or brunch. The delicate flavor of cream cheese combined with the punchy flavor of smoked salmon goes perfectly with the fragrant herbs and sharp onion flavor.

Time: 10 minutes

Serving Size:

1 serving

Ingredients:

- ½ tsp basil (dried or fresh)
- 2 tsp cream cheese
- ⅛ cup red onion (chopped)
- ¼ cup salmon (smoked)
- 1 flour tortilla (low-carb)
- arugula
- black pepper

Directions:

1. Warm up the tortilla in the microwave or oven.
2. In a bowl, combine the basil, cream cheese, and a pinch of pepper then spread onto the warmed tortilla.
3. Top with the salmon, onion, and a handful of arugula.
4. Roll up the tortilla and serve.

Cheese and Mushroom Frittata

In Italy, this is known as the "open-faced omelet." Frittatas are quick and easy to make, and they're extremely versatile too. You can enjoy them at any meal and use different ingredients for the filling. For this recipe, you will use creamy cheese and mushroom to complement the eggs for a scrumptious keto breakfast.

Time: 40 minutes

Serving Size: 4 servings

Ingredients for the frittata:

- ½ tsp black pepper
- 1 tsp salt
- 1 tbsp parsley (fresh)
- ½ cup butter
- ½ cup greens of choice
- 1 cup cheddar cheese (shredded)
- 1 cup keto-friendly mayonnaise
- 2 cups mushrooms (sliced)
- 6 scallions (chopped)
- 10 medium eggs

Ingredients for the sauce:

- ¼ tsp black pepper
- ½ tsp salt
- 1 tbsp white wine vinegar

- 4 tbsp olive oil

Directions:

1. Preheat your oven to 350°F and grease a baking dish with butter.
2. In a bowl, combine all of the sauce ingredients, mix well, and set aside.
3. In a pan, add the butter and mushrooms on medium-high heat and sauté until golden.
4. Turn the heat down and add the chopped scallions, parsley, salt, and pepper. Continue cooking for about 1 more minute then take the pan off the heat.
5. In a separate bowl, combine the cheese, mayonnaise, and eggs then mix well. You may also add a pinch of salt and pepper.
6. Add the cooked veggies and mix until well-incorporated. Pour the mixture into the baking dish you have prepared.
7. Place the baking dish in the oven and bake the frittata for about 30 to 40 minutes.
8. Take the baking dish out of the oven and allow the frittata to cool for about 5 minutes. Serve with the fresh greens and the sauce.

Oat Buttermilk Pancakes

Once you sink your teeth into these pancakes, you might not believe that they are low-carb. They're easy to make and they store well too. If you're craving for a pancake breakfast, you don't have to quash that craving because this recipe will save the day. You can also pair these pancakes with fruits or bacon depending on your own preference.

Time: 15 minutes

Serving Size: 5 servings

Ingredients:

- ½ tsp salt
- 2 tsp baking powder
- 4 tsp keto-friendly sweetener (powdered)
- 1 tbsp coconut oil
- ½ cup almond flour
- ½ cup oat fiber
- 1 cup buttermilk
- 4 medium eggs

Directions:

1. In a bowl, combine the baking powder, sweetener, almond flour, and oat fiber, then mix well.
2. Whisk in the eggs, oil, and buttermilk until all the ingredients are well-combined.
3. Heat butter or oil on a griddle and pour the batter into it.
4. Cook the pancakes for a few minutes on each side.
5. Transfer the cooked pancakes on serving plates, top with butter, and other toppings of choice.

Chocolate Chia Pudding

Chia pudding is another versatile recipe that you can enjoy for breakfast, dessert, or a snack, depending on the flavor you make. This particular recipe has a lovely chocolate flavor, and it only requires five ingredients. Aside from being keto- and diabetes-friendly, this dish is also gluten-free and vegan.

Time: 5 minutes (chilling time not included)

Serving Size: 2 servings

Ingredients:

- ¾ tsp sea salt
- 4 tbsp keto-friendly sweetener
- ½ cup chia seeds
- 1-⅓ cup almond milk (unsweetened)
- ⅓ cup of cocoa powder

Directions:

1. Sift the cocoa powder to give you a smoother texture without lumps.
2. In a bowl, combine all of the ingredients and whisk until you get a smooth, well-incorporated

mixture.

3. Pour the mixture into an airtight container and place in the refrigerator for a minimum of 1 hour. The longer you keep the pudding in the refrigerator, the firmer it becomes.

4. Before serving, garnish with whipped cream and your choice of fresh fruit.

Chapter 5: Keto Lunch Recipes for Type 2 Diabetes

Next up are some healthy lunch recipes. The great thing about these recipes is that they are easy to do, and you can enjoy them for dinner too. When you are following the keto diet, it's important to count your macros. Plan your meal combinations well so that you are able to meet your daily macros requirement – no more, no less. If this is your first time to cook on keto, starting off with these recipes will show you how easy it is to cook your own healthy meals at home.

Crustless Broccoli Quiche with Cheddar

Putting cheese and broccoli together makes for a healthy and tasty meal combination. This is a low-carb quiche sans the crust that's perfect for a light lunch or dinner. It takes less than an hour to make

– and even less to devour because it just tastes so good!

Time: 50 minutes

Serving Size: 6 servings

Ingredients:

- ⅛ tsp black pepper
- ¾ tsp kosher salt
- 1 tbsp water
- ¼ cup half & half cream
- ⅔ cup milk
- 1 cup cheddar cheese (grated)
- 3 cups broccoli florets (chopped)
- 5 large eggs
- nutmeg (freshly grated)
- cooking spray

Directions:

1. Preheat your oven to 350°F and grease a pie dish with cooking spray.
2. In a bowl, combine the water and broccoli florets and steam in the microwave for about 2 to 3 minutes until they are crisp and tender.
3. Transfer the broccoli into the pie dish and spread out evenly.
4. Top with the cheddar cheese and set aside.

5. In a bowl, combine the pepper, salt, half & half, milk, eggs, and a pinch of nutmeg then whisk well.
6. Pour the mixture over the layer of cheese and use a spatula to spread out evenly.
7. Place the pie dish in the oven and bake the quiche for about 35 to 40 minutes.
8. Take the pie dish out of the oven and allow the quiche to cool slightly before slicing.

Nicoise Tuna Salad

This is an interesting take on the classic Nicoise salad as it contains mustard and parsley dressing that gives a pleasant kick to it. This is a hearty and healthy lunch option that's easy to put together – perfect when you're always on the go. The best part is that even if you eat a huge portion of this salad, you won't be consuming a lot of calories, but you will still feel full for a long time!

Time: 15 minutes

Serving Size: 1 serving

Ingredients:

- ½ tsp black pepper
- ½ tsp Dijon mustard
- 1 tsp balsamic vinegar
- 1 tsp olive oil
- ¼ cup broccoli (steamed, diced)
- ¼ cup green beans (steamed)
- ½ cup cucumber (sliced)
- 2 cups baby spinach (washed, drained)
- ½ red bell pepper (diced)
- 1 egg (boiled, cooled, cut into bite-sized pieces)

- 1 ahi tuna steak
- 1 radish (sliced)
- 3 black olives (sliced)
- parsley (fresh, chopped)

Directions:

1. Season the tuna steak with pepper all over.
2. In a pan, add some oil and the seasoned tuna steak and cook over high heat for about 2 minutes per side.
3. In a bowl, add the spinach, red pepper, egg, and cucumber then toss lightly.
4. Add the radish, beans, and olives then continue tossing to mix all the ingredients together.
5. Slice the cooked tuna and add it to the bowl.
6. In a separate bowl, combine the balsamic vinegar, mustard, olive oil, salt, and pepper then whisk well.
7. Add the parsley to the vinaigrette and continue whisking to incorporate.
8. Drizzle the vinaigrette over your salad before serving.

Salmon-Stuffed Avocados

Aside from the perfect combination of smoked salmon and avocado, this dish doesn't require any cooking. It's creamy, smoky, and makes for a perfectly quick and luxurious lunch. You can also serve it as an appetizer or enjoy it as a light dinner. It's keto-friendly, delicious, and filled with healthy fats.

Time: 5 minutes

Serving Size: 2 servings

Ingredients:

- ¾ cup sour cream
- ¾ cup smoked salmon
- 2 medium-sized avocados
- black pepper
- salt
- 2 tbsp lemon juice (optional)

Directions:

1. Cut the avocados in half and take the pits out.
2. Divide the sour cream equally among the four avocado halves and spoon into the hollow of each

half.

3. Top with the smoked salmon then season with a pinch of salt and pepper. You may also add lemon juice before serving if desired.

Chicken Pesto Wraps

This simple salad wrap is another on-the-go dish that you can whip up in no time. Using lettuce or cabbage leaves makes it perfect for the keto diet and for diabetes too. It stores well, and it's really tasty!

Time: 5 minutes

Serving Size: 6 servings

Ingredients for the salad:

- ⅓ cup celery (chopped)
- ½ cup keto-friendly mayonnaise
- 2 cups chicken (cooked, cubed)
- black pepper
- salt
- cabbage or lettuce leaves
- avocado slices (optional)
- cheese (shredded, optional)
- cucumber slices (optional)
- tomato slices (optional)

Ingredients for the basil pesto sauce:

- 2 tsp garlic (minced)

- 3 tbsp pecans (toasted, cooled)
- ¼ cup olive oil
- 2 cups basil leaves

Directions:

1. In a blender, combine all the basil pesto ingredients and blend until you get a smooth consistency.
2. In a bowl, combine the chicken, basil pesto, celery, mayonnaise, and a pinch of salt and pepper, then stir well to combine.
3. Assemble the wraps. Start by scooping the chicken salad on a cabbage or lettuce leaf. Add any of the optional ingredients if desired before rolling up.

Hearty Spinach Rolls

These spinach rolls are filling, savory, and have the perfect spicy kick! This recipe is keto- and diabetes-friendly and it's also suitable for vegetarians. Spinach is one of the healthiest vegetables out there which is why you should try incorporating it into your meals more often. Here's one lunch recipe that will make you keep coming back for more.

Time: 55 minutes

Serving Size: 2 servings

Ingredients:

- ¼ tsp chili flakes
- 1 tsp black pepper
- 1 tsp curry powder
- 1 tsp salt
- ¼ cup carrot (grated)
- ¼ cup mozzarella cheese (shredded)
- ⅓ cup onion (finely chopped)
- ½ cup cottage cheese
- ¾ cup parsley (finely chopped)
- 2 cups spinach leaves (fresh)

- 1 garlic clove (minced)
- 3 eggs
- cooking spray

Directions:

1. Preheat your oven to 400°F and grease a baking sheet using the cooking spray.
2. In a bowl, combine the spinach, mozzarella, garlic, half of the salt and pepper, and 2 eggs then mix until well-incorporated.
3. Pour the mixture on the baking sheet and spread it evenly.
4. Place the baking sheet in the oven and bake the spinach mixture for about 15 minutes.
5. Take the baking sheet out of the oven and set it aside to cool.
6. In a skillet, add some oil and the onions then cook over medium heat for about 1 minute.
7. Add the parsley and carrots, mix well, and allow to simmer for 2 more minutes.
8. Add the curry powder, chili flakes, the other half of the salt and pepper, cottage cheese then mix until well-incorporated.
9. Take the skillet off the heat then add the remaining egg.
10. Mix all the ingredients together well then pour the mixture on the cooled spinach mixture.
11. Spread evenly being careful not to spread too close to the edges so the mixture doesn't spill out.

12. Roll up the baked spinach carefully and reposition on the baking sheet.
13. Place the baking sheet back in the oven and bake for about 25 minutes.
14. Take the baking sheet out of the oven and allow the spinach roll to cool for about 10 minutes before slicing and serving.

Chicken Thighs with Garlic and Mushrooms

This ravishing dish is so creamy and buttery that you might feel guilty about eating it. Of course, it also happens to be a guilt-free keto-friendly meal that you can enjoy with a fresh side dish like a green salad. Level up your keto menu by whipping up this dish for yourself to keep you motivated to stick with this unique diet.

Time: 20 minutes

Serving Size: 4 servings

Ingredients:

- ½ tsp rosemary (dried)
- 1 tsp garlic powder
- 1 tsp onion powder
- 1 tsp thyme (dried)
- 2 tbsp olive oil
- 4 tbsp butter
- ¼ cup parmesan cheese (grated)
- 1-¼ cups crème fraiche
- 4 cups mushrooms (roughly chopped)
- 1-½ lbs chicken thighs (boneless)
- 3 garlic cloves (minced)
- black pepper
- salt

Directions:

1. In a pan, heat the butter over medium heat.
2. Add the garlic and cook until golden.
3. Add the mushrooms and cook until tender and soft. Season with salt and pepper.
4. Transfer the mushrooms to a bowl then set aside.
5. In a bowl, combine all the spices and mix well.
6. Coat the chicken thighs with the spice mixture

evenly.

7. Add some olive oil to the same pan along with the chicken thighs then fry for about 6 to 7 minutes per side.

8. Once cooked, take the chicken thighs off the pan and keep warm.

9. Still in the same pan, add the parmesan and crème fraiche.

10. Mix well, bring to a boil, turn the heat down, and allow to simmer for about 5 minutes as you stir constantly. Season with salt and pepper as you continue stirring until the sauce thickens.

11. Place the chicken thighs back into the pan along with the cooked mushrooms and serve while hot.

Huevos Rancheros

This keto-friendly twist on the Mexican classic combines elements of "shakshuka," the classic Tunisian dish. It's saucy, a bit spicy, and oh-so-delicious. It's a filling meal you can enjoy for lunch or dinner so you can reach your target macros count. And it's easy to make too!

Time: 45 minutes

Serving Size: 4 servings

Ingredients:

- ½ tsp salt
- ½ tsp cumin (ground)
- 1 tbsp hot sauce
- 2 tbsp olive oil
- ½ onion (chopped)
- ¾ cup black beans (canned, drained)
- ¾ cup tomatoes (crushed or diced)
- 2 garlic cloves (chopped)
- 4 eggs
- avocado (sliced, for topping)
- cilantro leaves (for topping)

- feta cheese (crumbled, for topping)
- radishes (sliced, for topping)

Directions:

1. Preheat your oven to 375°F.
2. In an oven-proof skillet, add some oil along with the garlic and onion over medium heat. Sauté until the onion turns golden and starts softening, about 6 minutes.
3. Add the hot sauce and cumin then continue to sauté for a few more seconds.
4. Add the beans, tomatoes, and salt then turn the heat down to medium-low.
5. Stir occasionally while cooking for about 15 more minutes until the sauce thickens.
6. Using the back of a spoon, press down gently on the sauce to make a small well. Crack one of the eggs into it gently. Repeat with the rest of the eggs.
7. Place the skillet in the oven and bake the dish between 7 to 15 minutes depending on how you like your eggs cooked.
8. Take the skillet out of the oven and serve while hot.

Creamy Broccoli Casserole

This creamy and rich keto-friendly casserole can be a light lunch or an addition to your meal. It's the perfect comfort food that you can make in a jiffy. The cheese sauce smothers the crisp broccoli and the whole casserole is roasted to make a mouthwatering dish to share with the whole family.

Time: 45 minutes

Serving Size: 6 servings

Ingredients:

- ½ tsp black pepper
- 1 tsp basil (dried)
- 1 tsp sea salt
- 1 tbsp yellow mustard
- 2 tbsp butter (unsalted)
- ¼ cup mozzarella cheese (grated)
- ½ cup heavy cream
- 1 cup cream cheese
- 1 cup white cheddar cheese (grated)
- 3-¾ cups broccoli (cut into florets)
- 2 garlic cloves (minced)

Directions:

1. Preheat your oven to 350°F and grease a casserole dish.
2. In a pot, combine the cream, butter, and cream cheese over medium heat. Stir the mixture occasionally until all of the ingredients have melted and are well-combined.
3. Turn the heat down to low and add the pepper, salt, basil, mustard, garlic, and grated cheeses.
4. Continue mixing until the cheeses have melted

completely and you get a creamy and smooth mixture.

5. Add the broccoli florets to the casserole dish and spread out evenly.

6. Pour the sauce over the broccoli and mix well to coat all the florets evenly.

7. Spread the coated broccoli in a single layer and top with more grated mozzarella cheese.

8. Place the casserole dish in the oven and bake the casserole for about 30 minutes.

9. Take the casserole dish out of the oven and allow the casserole to cool for about 10 minutes before serving.

Chapter 6: Keto Dinner Recipes for Type 2 Diabetes

Dinner is the time for you to complete your macros requirement for the day. Unless you are meal planning (which is highly recommended on the ketogenic diet), it's important to count your calories at each meal, especially in terms of the fats, protein, and carbs you have already consumed for breakfast, lunch, and even if you had an afternoon snack. If you had filling meals throughout the day, then you should consume a light dinner. Conversely, if you had light meals throughout the day, then you may treat yourself to a healthy and hearty dinner. Following the keto diet successfully is all about finding the right balance each and every day.

Baked BLT Avocado Eggs

These baked avocado eggs make the perfect dinner (or lunch). This dish is low in carbs, high in healthy fats, and will keep you feeling full for a long time. They're easy to make, take less than an hour, but are so satisfying to eat.

Time: 25 minutes

Serving Size: 4 servings

Ingredients:

- ¼ cup bacon (cooked, chopped)
- ¼ cup lettuce leaves (shredded)
- 2 medium avocados
- 4 cherry tomatoes (cut into four)
- 4 medium eggs
- black pepper
- salt

Directions:

1. Preheat your oven to 375°F and line a baking sheet with parchment paper.
2. Cut both avocados in half and take the pit out.
3. Make the hole left by the pit bigger by scooping out some of the flesh as needed. Remove just

enough for an egg to fit inside.

4. Place the prepared avocado halves on the baking sheet.
5. Crack the eggs into each of the holes you have made then season with salt and pepper.
6. Top the eggs with bacon and cherry tomatoes.
7. Place the baking sheet in the oven and bake the avocados for about 15 to 18 minutes depending on how you like your eggs.
8. Take the baking sheet out of the oven and top each of the avocado halves with shredded lettuce leaves before serving.

Herb Marinated Turkey Breast Bites

This recipe is quick, healthy, and oh-so-satisfying to eat. It has a perfect combination of flavors with minimum work required. This recipe takes boring turkey breasts and elevates them to an absolutely delicious dish. With the strong flavors, you don't even have to add condiments or sauces that may contain extra carbs.

Time: 50 minutes

Serving Size: 1 serving

Ingredients:

- ¼ tsp basil (dried)
- ¼ tsp black pepper
- ¼ tsp garlic powder
- ¼ tsp thyme
- 1 tsp olive oil
- 1-½ balsamic vinegar
- ½ cup turkey breast (cubed)

Directions:

1. In a bowl, combine the pepper, basil, thyme, olive oil, and balsamic vinegar then mix well.
2. Place the cubed turkey breast in the bowl, toss to coat, and set aside for at least 30 minutes to marinate.
3. In a skillet, heat some oil and add the marinated turkey breast cubes over medium heat. Fry for about 5 to 8 minutes until fully cooked. Serve while hot.

Mashed Cauliflower with Spinach

This dish will satisfy your mashed potato craving sans the carbs – and guilt. Adding spinach to the dish makes it healthier and tastier too. While regular mashed cauliflower already serves as an excellent side dish, this recipe improves it by adding more color and flavor. Plus, you can enjoy this on its own as a filling dinner.

Time: 30 minutes

Serving Size: 8 servings

Ingredients:

- ¼ tsp dill weed (dried)
- 1-½ tsp onion (dried, minced)
- ½ cup butter
- 1 cup cheddar cheese (grated)
- 1 cup sour cream
- 1-¼ cup spinach (chopped, cooked, drained)
- 1 medium cauliflower head (chopped)
- salt

Directions:

1. In a pot, bring water to a boil. Add the

cauliflower, cook for about 6 minutes then drain.

2. In a food processor, combine the cauliflower and butter then pulse until well-blended.

3. Add the dill weed, dried onion, sour cream, spinach, and a pinch of salt then continue pulsing until well-combined.

4. Transfer the mixture into a greased casserole dish and top with cheddar cheese.

5. Place the casserole dish in the oven and bake at 350°F for about 20 minutes.

6. Take the casserole dish out of the oven and allow to cool slightly before serving.

Spiced Shrimp Salad

If you love spicy food, then this is the perfect recipe for you. This piquant salad will awaken your taste buds along with the rest of your senses. It has smooth avocado, crunchy cucumber, and hot shrimp combined with a tasty garlic and ginger dressing. Perfect!

Time: 5 minutes

Serving Size: 2 servings

Ingredients for the salad:

- 2 tsp chili powder
- 3 tbsp olive oil
- ¼ cup baby spinach (washed, drained)
- ⅔ cup cucumber (chopped)
- 1-¼ cup shrimp (peeled)
- ½ lime (juiced)
- 1 garlic clove (pressed)
- 2 medium avocados
- cilantro (fresh)
- 2 tbsp hazelnuts (optional, chopped)

Ingredients for the dressing:

- ½ tbsp tamari soy sauce
- 1 tbsp ginger (fresh, minced)
- ¼ cup avocado oil
- ½ garlic clove (pressed)
- ½ lime (juiced)
- black pepper
- salt

Directions:

1. Cut the avocados in half and take the pit out.
2. Scoop out pieces of avocado using a spoon then slice.
3. Drizzle with lime juice and season with salt.
4. On a plate, combine the avocado, cucumber, and spinach. Season with salt and toss lightly.
5. In a pan, add some oil along with the chili powder

and garlic then fry until fragrant.

6. Add the shrimps and fry for 2 to 3 minutes on each side. Season with salt and pepper.

7. Place the shrimp over the vegetables then sprinkle with cilantro and nuts, if desired.

8. In an immersion blender, combine all the dressing ingredients.

9. Blend until smooth then drizzle over the salad before serving.

10.

Turkey Meatloaf Muffins

Turkey meatloaf? Have you ever heard of such a thing? Well, it does exist, and it's completely keto-friendly. These cheesy turkey meatloaf muffins will surely satisfy your taste buds each time you eat them. And since they come in muffin form, you don't have to slice them or think about portion sizes.

Time: 1 hour

Serving Size: 12 muffins

Ingredients:

- ½ tsp oregano (dried)
- 1 tsp salt
- 1 tbsp coconut oil
- 1 tbsp Worcestershire sauce
- 2 tbsp parsley (fresh)
- ½ cup onion (chopped)
- ¾ cup pork rinds (crushed)
- 1 cup mozzarella cheese (grated)

- 2 lbs turkey (ground)
- 2 large eggs
- 4 garlic cloves (finely chopped)
- ketchup (optional, sugar-free)

Directions:

1. Preheat your oven to 350°F and use coconut oil to grease a muffin pan.
2. In a large bowl, combine all the ingredients then mix until everything is well-incorporated.
3. Spoon the meatloaf mixture into the muffin pan.
4. Place the muffin pan in the oven and bake the muffins for about 55 minutes.
5. Take the muffin pan out of the oven and allow the muffins to cool slightly before serving. Serve with ketchup for dipping if desired.

Tuna Poke

This is a classic Hawaiian method of preparing raw tuna (or other types of fish) with spices, sesame oil, and soy sauce. Basically, it's the Hawaiian's version of sushi. This is another easy recipe that takes only 10 minutes to put together. If you're searching for a quick dinner option, this is the one.

Time: 20 minutes

Serving Size: 2 servings

Ingredients:

- 1 tbsp chili garlic sauce
- 1 tbsp sesame oil
- 2 tbsp sesame seeds
- 2 tbsp soy sauce (low-sodium)
- ½ lb Ahi tuna (sushi-grade)
- 1 medium avocado (cubed)
- 2 scallions (chopped)

Directions:

1. Rinse the tuna then cut it into bite-sized pieces.
2. In a bowl, combine the chili garlic sauce, sesame oil, soy sauce, scallions, and half of the sesame

seeds then mix well.

3. Add the tuna pieces and continue mixing to coat evenly.

4. Chill in the refrigerator for about 10 minutes allowing the flavors to mix and get absorbed by the tuna (you may skip this step if you want).

5. Before serving, add the avocado cubes and mix gently. Sprinkle with the rest of the sesame seeds and serve.

Grilled Vegetables Platter

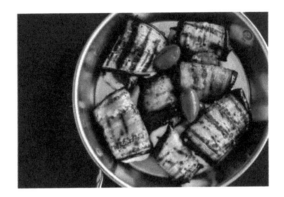

Get a huge serving of vegetables in one meal with this Mediterranean-inspired masterpiece. This dish is a fresh combination of grilled veggies, nuts, cheese, and olives that make for a scrumptious keto-friendly dinner. The drizzle of lemon and olive oil adds flavor to it and make the perfect finishing touch.

Time: 20 minutes

Serving Size: 2 servings

Ingredients:

- 2 tbsp almonds

- ⅛ cup leafy greens
- ¼ cup olive oil
- ½ cup crème fraiche
- ⅔ cup cheddar cheese (sliced)
- ⅓ eggplant (sliced lengthwise)
- ½ lemon (juiced)
- ½ zucchini (sliced lengthwise)
- 10 black olives (sliced)
- black pepper
- salt

Directions:

1. Season the zucchini and eggplant slices with salt then set them aside for about 10 minutes.
2. Preheat your oven and set it to broil then use parchment paper to line a baking sheet.
3. Using paper towels, pat the zucchini and eggplant slices dry.
4. Place the zucchini and eggplant slices on the baking sheet, brush with olive oil, then season with pepper.
5. Place the baking sheet in the oven and broil the zucchini and eggplant slices for about 15 to 20 minutes.
6. Take the baking sheet out of the oven and place the zucchini and eggplant slices on a serving platter.
7. Add the almonds, olives, cheese slices, and leafy greens to the plate along with the crème fraiche

on the side.

8. Drizzle the zucchini and eggplant slices with lemon juice and olive oil and serve.

Greek Salad

This incredible low-carb salad includes "zoodles" – a fun and healthy way to include zucchini in your meal. This is another simple dinner recipe that's easy to put together in a matter of 5 minutes. It's fresh, crunchy, delicious, and is the perfect light meal to end your day.

Time: 5 minutes

Serving Size: 6 servings

Ingredients:

- ⅛ tsp black pepper
- ¼ tsp sea salt
- ½ tsp oregano (dried)
- 3 tbsp red wine vinegar
- 6 tbsp olive oil
- ½ cup feta cheese (crumbled)
- ½ cup Kalamata olives (pitted, sliced)
- 1 cup tomatoes (cubed)
- 1 green bell pepper (chopped)
- 1 medium zucchini (spiralized)
- 2 cucumbers (peeled, sliced)
- 1 pepperoncino (optional, sliced)

- 8 slices of salami (optional)

Directions:

1. In a bowl, combine the pepper, salt, oregano, vinegar, and olive oil then whisk well.
2. In a separate bowl, combine the feta cheese, Kalamata olives, tomatoes, bell pepper, and cucumbers. Also, add the pepperoncino and salami slices if desired.
3. Add the dressing and toss lightly to coat all the ingredients evenly.
4. Place the spiralized zucchini on a serving plate, top with the salad, and serve.

Chapter 7: Keto Dessert Recipes for Type 2 Diabetes

Who says that you cannot have desserts while on keto – or if you suffer from type 2 diabetes? While you should be careful when it comes to sugar when you have this condition, this doesn't mean that you can never eat desserts again. The great thing about the ketogenic diet is that it has become so trendy and mainstream that manufacturers have started creating their own versions of keto-friendly sugar substitutes – which also happen to be suitable for diabetics too. Here are some simple keto dessert recipes for you to start with.

Pistachio and Pomegranate Bark

Chocolate is one of the most popular dessert choices. This versatile ingredient can be enjoyed on its own, and it comes in different variations. For this recipe, you will be using dark chocolate, which is healthier and more suitable for keto. This chocolate bark is combined with pomegranates and pistachios to make it healthier and more satisfying as a sweet treat after your meal.

Time: 20 minutes (chilling time not included)

Serving Size: 1 batch

Ingredients:

- ⅛ tsp sea salt
- ½ cup pistachios (raw, shelled, roughly chopped)
- ½ cup pomegranate seeds (drained)
- 2-⅓ cups dark chocolate (broken into small pieces)

Directions:

1. Use parchment paper to line a baking sheet then set aside.
2. In a skillet, add the pistachios over medium heat, cook for about 3 minutes then set aside to cool.
3. In a saucepan, bring some water to a boil over medium heat then reduce the heat to low allowing the water to simmer.
4. Place the chocolate in a heat-proof bowl then place the bowl on top of the saucepan.
5. Heat the chocolate for about 5 minutes to melt while you stir gently.

6. Pour the melted chocolate into the baking sheet then use a spatula to spread evenly all the way to the edges.
7. Sprinkle with pomegranate seeds and toasted pistachios.
8. Place the baking sheet in the refrigerator to chill for about 1 hour for the chocolate to set.
9. Break the chocolate bark into pieces then store in an airtight container.

Gingerbread Crème Brûlée

This recipe combines dreamy gingerbread with creamy custard for an indulgent yet healthy snack. It's an incredible keto dessert that finishes your meals off with a perfectly-spiced treat. This dish gives an interesting twist to a classic dessert that we all know and love.

Time: 30 minutes

Serving Size: 6 servings

Ingredients:

- ¼ tsp vanilla extract
- 2 tsp pumpkin pie spice
- 2 tbsp erythritol
- 1-¾ cups heavy whipping cream
- 4 eggs (yolks only)
- ½ clementine (optional)

Directions:

1. Preheat your oven to 360°F and add water to a baking dish.
2. In a saucepan, add the cream along with the vanilla extract, erythritol, and pumpkin pie spice, mix well, and bring to a boil.
3. In a bowl, add the egg yolks then pour the cream mixture a little bit at a time as you whisk continuously.
4. Pour the mixture into ramekins then place the ramekins in the baking dish with water.
5. Place the baking dish in the oven and bake for about 30 minutes.
6. Take the baking dish out of the oven and the ramekins out of the baking dish, and allow to cool.
7. Top each serving with one clementine segment before serving.

Protein Jelly Cheesecake

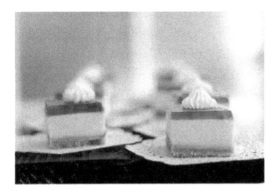

When you're craving for a heavier dessert to complete a light meal, look no further than this yummy cheesecake. Since it's almost completely made of protein, it also makes an excellent bedtime snack to leave you satisfied while feeding your muscles while you sleep. This low-carb cheesecake will satisfy your cravings without taking up all of your daily caloric requirements.

Time: 1 hour

Serving Size: 1 cheesecake

Ingredients:

- 1 tsp vanilla extract
- 1 tbsp keto-friendly sweetener (powdered)
- 1 cup cottage cheese

- 1 scoop protein powder (vanilla)
- 1 pack Jell-O (sugar-free, strawberry flavor)
- 2 eggs (whites only)
- water

Directions:

1. Preheat your oven to 325°F and grease a non-stick pan.
2. Follow the Jell-O packet instructions then place it in the freezer until almost set.
3. In a bowl, combine the egg whites and cottage cheese then blend until you get a smooth consistency.
4. Add the protein powder, vanilla extract, and sweetener then whisk until everything is well-incorporated.
5. Pour the batter into the non-stick pan.
6. Place the non-stick pan in the oven and bake the cake for about 25 minutes.
7. Turn your oven off with the cake still inside.
8. When the Jell-O is ready, pour it over the cooled cheesecake.
9. Place the cheesecake in the refrigerator to set for about 10 to 12 hours before serving.

Crunchy Berry Mousse

Experience incredible tastiness with this creative and creamy mousse recipe. It's simple, healthy, and it will surely wow your loved ones. It has fresh berries for flavor, pecans for texture, and lemon zest to balance everything out. This is a festive treat that you can enjoy at any time of the day.

Time: 10 minutes (chilling time not included)

Serving Size: 8 servings

Ingredients:

- ¼ tsp vanilla extract
- ¼ cup pecans (chopped)
- ½ cup raspberries (fresh, you can also use blueberries or strawberries)
- 2 cups heavy whipping cream
- ½ lemon (zest only)

Directions:

1. In a bowl, add the heavy cream and use a hand mixer to whip until you form soft peaks. Add the vanilla extract and lemon zest towards the end.
2. Add the nuts and berries then stir well to incorporate.
3. Cover the bowl with plastic food wrap then place in the refrigerator for a minimum of 3 hours before serving.

4.

Ice Box Peanut Butter Bars

These peanut butter bars are so yummy and addictive that you might have to restrain yourself from eating the whole batch when it's ready! These bars have a perfect combination of flavors from the healthy ingredients you use to make them. This is another easy dessert you can whip up in a jiffy.

Time: 30 minutes (freezing time not included)

Serving Size: 12 bars

Ingredients:

- ½ tsp vanilla extract
- 2 tbsp butter (unsalted)
- ¼ cup dark chocolate
- ½ cup peanut butter (natural, creamy)
- 1 cup Greek yogurt (vanilla)
- 3 bananas (ripe)
- 8 graham crackers

Directions:

1. Preheat your oven to 350°F and grease a baking dish.
2. In a Ziploc bag, add all the graham crackers then seal it.
3. Use your hands, a rolling pin or any other hard object to crush the crackers into crumbs.
4. In a microwave-safe bowl, add the butter, melt in the microwave, and cool for about 1 minute.
5. Add the crushed graham crackers and stir until well-combined.
6. Transfer the mixture into the baking dish and spread it all the way to the edges evenly using a spatula.

7. Place the baking dish in the oven and bake the crust for about 10 minutes.

8. Take the baking dish out of the oven and set aside to cool.

9. In a bowl, add the bananas and mash them.

10. In a separate bowl, combine the vanilla extract, Greek yogurt, and peanut butter, then stir well to combine.

11. Fold the bananas in gently until well-incorporated.

12. Pour the banana mixture over the crust.

13. Place the baking dish in the freezer for a minimum of 3 hours.

14. In a microwave-safe bowl, add the chocolate and melt in the microwave for about 1 minute stirring after 30 seconds.

15. Take the baking dish out of the freezer and drizzle the melted chocolate on top before slicing into bars.

Coconut and Strawberry Fat Bombs

These tasty fat bombs are so simple and easy to make. They require simple ingredients to give you a flavorful dessert that can also serve as a filling snack. They are energy powerhouses filled with healthy fats to give you energy and keep you feeling full until your next meal. The creamy coconut oil and coconut cream make the perfect base to imitate the richness and creaminess of strawberry cheesecake.

Time: 10 minutes (freezing time not included)

Serving Size: 20 fat bombs

Ingredients for the base:

- 1 tbsp lime juice
- ½ tsp keto-friendly sweetener (liquid)
- ½ cup coconut oil (melted)
- 1-½ cup coconut cream

Ingredients for the topping:

- ¼ cup strawberries (fresh, chopped)
- ½ cup coconut oil (melted)
- 5 - 8 drops keto-friendly sweetener (liquid)

•

Directions:

1. In a blender, add all the base ingredients then blend until you get a smooth texture.
2. Pour the mixture into a muffin pan until more than halfway full.
3. Place the muffin pan in the freezer for about 20 minutes.
4. In a blender, add all the topping ingredients then blend until you get a smooth texture.
5. Take the muffin pan out of the freezer and spoon one layer of the topping on top of the base.
6. Place the muffin pan in the refrigerator and chill overnight before serving.

Strawberry Granita

This semi-frozen dessert is healthy, refreshing, and oh-so-simple. It requires very few ingredients and you can even change the flavor by changing the main ingredient. This dessert is perfect for hot summer days after you have just enjoyed a heavy, fat-rich keto meal. You can also enjoy it as a snack for when the days become sweltering hot.

Time: 40 minutes (freezing time not included)

Serving Size: 6 servings

Ingredients:

- 1 tbsp lemon juice
- ¾ cup keto-friendly sweetener
- 1 cup of water
- 2 cups strawberries

Directions:

1. In a food processor, add the strawberries and purée.
2. Add the lemon juice, sweetener, and water then pulse until well-combined.
3. Pour the mixture into a baking pan and place in the freezer for about 30 minutes.
4. Take the baking pan out of the oven, use a fork to stir the mixture then return to the freezer for 2 more hours. Just take it out every 30 minutes to stir and break up large pieces.
5. When serving, garnish with a sprig of mint if desired.

Saffron Panna Cotta

This gorgeous dessert is simple, creamy, and elegant. It has a bright color that makes it look amazing – and one taste will make you realize that it tastes as amazing as it looks. This dessert is what keto dreams are made of, so learning how to make it will truly elevate your dessert-making skills.

Time: 10 minutes (chilling time not included)

Serving Size: 6 servings

Ingredients:

- ¼ tsp vanilla extract
- ½ tbsp gelatin (powdered, unflavored)
- 2 cups heavy whipping cream
- saffron
- water
- 1 tbsp almonds (optional, chopped)
- 1 tbsp honey (optional)
- 12 raspberries (optional, fresh)

Directions:

1. In a bowl, combine the gelatin powder with some water then set aside.
2. In a saucepan, combine the heavy cream, vanilla extract, and a pinch of honey over medium heat then bring to a boil. You may also add honey if desired.
3. Once boiling, turn the heat down to low and allow to simmer for a couple of minutes.
4. Take the saucepan off the heat, add the gelatin mixture, and stir well until dissolved.
5. Pour the mixture into ramekins, cover with plastic food wrap, and place in your refrigerator to chill

for a minimum of 2 hours.

6. If desired, add the almonds to a pan and cook for a couple of minutes until toasted.

7. Serve the panna cotta as is or top with toasted almonds and fresh raspberries.

Chapter 8: Keto Snack Recipes for Type 2 Diabetes

Finally, we have some healthy snack recipes. When you suffer from type 2 diabetes, you must make sure that your blood sugar levels don't drop too low – and this is where snacks come in. Enjoying healthy, keto- and diabetes-friendly snacks help stabilize your blood sugar and insulin levels without compromising your health. The great thing about some of these recipes – particularly the sweet ones – is that you can have them for dessert as well. Mix and match all the recipes you have learned from this book so you can come up with a healthy meal plan each day that allows you to consume all the calories and macros you need to achieve and maintain ketosis.

Chocolate Fat Bombs

If you enjoy chocolates, you would be happy to know that it's possible to eat this sweet treat while on keto – as long as you choose your chocolate treats well. Fat bombs are very popular on the keto diet because they contain a lot of healthy fats, which help you reach your diet goals. This recipe may become one of your favorites once you get a bite of these fat bombs.

Time: 25 minutes

Serving Size: 12 fat bombs

Ingredients:

- 1 tsp vanilla extract
- 2 tbsp keto-friendly sweetener
- 2 tbsp heavy cream
- 5 tbsp peanut butter (natural, chunky)
- 6 tbsp hemp seeds (shelled)
- ¼ cup of cocoa powder (unsweetened)
- ½ cup of coconut oil (unrefined)
- coconut (optional, shredded)

Directions:

1. In a bowl, combine the hemp seeds, cocoa powder, and peanut butter then mix well.
2. Add the coconut oil and continue mixing until you get a pasty consistency.
3. Add the vanilla extract, sweetener, and heavy cream then continue mixing until everything is well-incorporated.
4. Use your hands to scoop the mixture and roll into balls.
5. Roll the balls in shredded coconut if desired.
6. Line a baking tray with parchment paper and place the fat bombs.

7. Place the baking tray in the refrigerator for at least 30 minutes before serving.

Oven-Baked Brie

This dish is creamy, comforting, elegant, and is a filling keto diet snack. Enjoy the lovely flavor of Brie which has been warmed paired with toasted nuts and fresh herbs. You'll enjoy this snack so much that you may want to serve it at your next party! It also serves as a satisfying dessert too.

Time: 10 minutes

Serving Size: 4 servings

Ingredients:

- 1 tbsp olive oil
- 1 tbsp rosemary (fresh, coarsely chopped)
- ¼ cup walnuts (coarsely chopped)
- 1-¼ cup Brie cheese
- 1 garlic clove (minced)
- black pepper
- salt

Directions:

1. Preheat your oven to 400°F and line a baking sheet with parchment paper.
2. Place the Brie on the baking sheet.
3. In a bowl, combine the herbs, nuts, garlic, and olive oil together. Season with salt and pepper then mix well.
4. Pour the mixture over the cheese.
5. Place the baking sheet in the oven and bake for about 10 minutes.
6. Take the baking sheet out of the oven and serve warm.

Banana and Raspberry Mousse

This high-protein mousse is an excellent snack when you need a boost of protein to complete your macros count. It has a silky and thick consistency sans the unhealthy ingredients you would typically find in a dish as indulgent as this one. This mousse is versatile too because you can use other berries as a substitute for the raspberries.

Time: 5 minutes

Serving Size: 1 serving

Ingredients:

- 1 tbsp keto-friendly sweetener
- ⅓ cup raspberries (frozen)
- ¼ cup banana (frozen)
- 2 medium eggs (whites only)
- raspberries (optional, fresh)

Directions:

1. In a bowl, combine the sweetener and egg whites, then use a hand mixer to blend for about 2 minutes until firm.
2. Add the raspberries and bananas then continue

137

blending until you get a smooth, pink-colored consistency.

3. Spoon the mousse into serving bowls and top with fresh berries if desired before serving.

Choco-Avocado Pudding

Chocolate and avocado are a match made in heaven. It's a creamy and healthy comfort food that you can indulge in when you're craving for a sweet snack. This rich, chocolatey mousse. Avocados are frequently featured in keto recipes because they add a lot of beneficial nutrients to dishes both sweet or savory.

Time: 10 minutes (chilling time not included)

Serving Size: 6 servings

Ingredients:

- 1 tsp vanilla extract
- ¼ cup almond milk (unsweetened, divided)
- ¼ cup chocolate chips (semi-sweet)
- ¼ cup of cocoa powder
- 1 medium avocado (ripe)
- almonds or strawberries (optional, for topping)

Directions:

1. Slice the avocado in half, scoop the flesh out, and add to a blender.
2. In a microwave-safe bowl, add the chocolate chips and melt in the microwave.
3. Add the melted chocolate to the blender along with the cocoa powder, vanilla extract, and half of the almond milk.
4. Blend all of the ingredients until you get a smooth consistency.
5. Pour the mixture into a bowl and place in the refrigerator to chill for about 30 minutes.
6. Before serving, top with almonds or strawberries if desired.

Lemon Tofu Crème

This sugar-free, gluten-free, and keto-friendly snack is suitable for vegans too. You can enjoy this on its own or use it as a topping for desserts and other sweet dishes. You can use extra firm or firm tofu for this recipe depending on your preferences. But the best way to enjoy this snack – and make it more filling – is by pairing it with fresh fruits and chopped nuts.

Time: 6 minutes

Serving Size: 4 servings

Ingredients:

- 1 tsp keto-friendly sweetener
- 1 tsp lemon zest
- ¼ cup lemon juice (fresh)
- 1 cup tofu (firm or extra firm, drained)
- 1 large lemon (zest and juice)
- chopped nuts (optional)
- fresh fruits (optional)

Directions:

1. Use paper towels to pat the tofu as dry as possible.

2. In a food processor, combine all of the ingredients and blend until you get a smooth mixture.
3. Transfer the mixture to a bowl and chill in the refrigerator.
4. Before serving, top with chopped nuts and fresh fruits if desired.

Peanut Butter Cookies

These low-carb, sugar-free cookies can be enjoyed at any time of the day. Whether you're craving for a morning or afternoon snack, you can munch on these deliciously simple peanut butter cookies. They're so simple because they only require five ingredients to make! Eating one or two of these cookies for your snack won't ruin your diet either.

Time: 20 minutes

Serving Size: 12 cookies

Ingredients:

- ½ tsp baking soda
- ½ tsp vanilla extract
- ⅔ cup erythritol (powdered)

- 1 cup peanut butter (sugar-free, smooth)
- 1 large egg

Directions:

1. Preheat your oven to 350°F and line a cookie sheet with parchment paper.
2. In a bowl, combine all the ingredients and mix well until you form a dough.
3. Scoop 2 tablespoons of the dough then shape the dough into balls with your hands.
4. Place the dough balls on the cookie sheet then use a fork to press down on the center of each cookie to make them flat.
5. Place the cookie sheet in the oven and bake the cookies for about 12 to 15 minutes.
6. Take the cookie sheet out of the oven and allow the cookies to cool for about 25 minutes.
7. Transfer the cookies to a cooling rack and allow the cookies to cool for 15 more minutes before serving.

Coconut Pudding

Are you looking for a traditional pudding recipe that's low in carbs? Then this is the recipe for you. This is a creamy pudding with a lovely coconut flavor that comes from the perfect cream cheese and coconut milk combination. It takes a mere 15 minutes to make but you will be enjoying its taste for longer than that.

Time: 15 minutes

Serving Size: 4 servings

Ingredients:

- ½ tsp vanilla extract
- 1 tsp coconut extract
- ¼ cup keto-friendly sweetener (granular)
- ½ cup coconut (unsweetened, shredded)
- ½ cup coconut cream
- ½ cup of coconut milk
- ½ cup cream cheese (cut into small pieces)
- 1 egg (beaten)

Directions:

1. In a microwave-safe bowl, combine half of the coconut cream with the sweetener, vanilla extract, coconut extract, and shredded coconut.

2. Place the bowl in the microwave, heat on high for 1 minute then set aside.

3. In a separate bowl, combine the rest of the cream with the egg, beat until well-combined, and set aside.

4. In a saucepan, combine the cream cheese and coconut milk then cook over medium heat until all the cream cheese pieces have melted.

5. Add the mixture you heated in the microwave then continue cooking for about 2 minutes.

6. Add the egg mixture then continue cooking while stirring constantly until it thickens.

7. Pour the mixture into small baking dishes and allow to cool to room temperature.

8. Once cool, chill in the refrigerator for about 30 minutes before serving.

Apples with Cinnamon and Vanilla Sauce

Once you get a taste of this snack, you will be craving for it over and over again. It has a creamy sauce with spices that will warm you up pleasantly. While the sauce pairs perfectly with the cinnamon apples, you can also pair it with other snacks and desserts because it's just so versatile!

Time: 20 minutes

Serving Size: 6 servings

Ingredients for the sauce:

- ½ tsp vanilla extract
- 2 tbsp butter
- 2-½ cups heavy whipping cream
- 1 medium egg (yolk only)
- 1 piece of star anise (optional)

Ingredients for the apples:

- 1 tsp cinnamon (ground)
- 3 tbsp butter

- 3 Granny Smith apples (or other tart, firm type of apple)

Directions:

1. In a saucepan, combine the vanilla extract, butter, about ¼ of the heavy whipping cream, and the star anise, if desired, over medium heat.
2. Allow the mixture to come to a boil then turn down the heat to low.
3. Allow to simmer for about 5 minutes while stirring constantly until it turns creamy.
4. Take the saucepan off the heat, scoop out the star anise, and transfer the mixture to a bowl.
5. Add the egg yolk into the heated mixture while you whisk vigorously.
6. Place the bowl in the refrigerator to cool down completely.
7. In a separate bowl, add the rest of the heavy whipping cream and whisk until you form soft peaks.
8. Fold in the chilled sauce.
9. Place the mixture back into the refrigerator for at least 30 more minutes.
10. Rinse the apples, core them, and cut them into thin slices.
11. In a pan, melt the butter over medium heat and add the apple slices.
12. Cook the apple slices until golden brown in color. Towards the end of the cooking process, add the

cinnamon and toss lightly to coat all of the apple slices.

13. Serve warm and top with the chilled vanilla sauce.

Conclusion: Living the Keto Lifestyle with Type 2 Diabetes

Living with type 2 diabetes isn't an easy thing. When you are diagnosed with this condition, you may need to search for ways to make your life easier. For this condition, one of the most difficult things to deal with is your diet. But if you want to make this condition easier to manage, you need to make some changes in your lifestyle and diet – if only there were standard rules you can follow, right?

Well, if you choose to start the ketogenic diet, you may discover that changing your diet for the benefit of your condition isn't that difficult – after all, the ketogenic diet already comes with its own set of rules. This high-fat, low-carb, moderate-protein diet is ideal for anyone who suffers from type 2 diabetes – unless you are undergoing insulin therapy.

Since you are suffering from a medical condition, it's best to consult with your doctor first before you go keto. Fortunately, you have already learned all the fundamental information about this diet through this book. With all this information and knowledge, you can have a more enriching conversation with your doctor about following the diet to manage your condition more effectively.

At the beginning of this book, you learned all about type 2 diabetes. Learning more about your condition will help you understand it better – and it also helps you see why keto is beneficial for type 2 diabetes. Then we moved on to the ketogenic diet and how to follow it – from what foods to eat, what foods to avoid, and some easy and practical tips to employ for following the keto diet while suffering from type 2 diabetes.

Next up was the chapter about cooking on keto. Here, you learned the importance of cooking your own meals as this helps you follow through with the diet long-term. This chapter also included tips for basic keto ingredients and some helpful tips for meal planning.

The next part of the book focused on easy, healthy, tasty, and simple recipes you can start making in your kitchen right now. We started with breakfast recipes then moved on to lunch, dinner, dessert, and snack recipes, all of which are keto-friendly and suitable for your condition. From beginning to end, this book provided you with everything you need to start your keto journey. If there is one thing you should have taken from this book, it's the knowledge that following keto doesn't have to be a challenge and you should start this diet now in order to experience all the benefits it has to offer.

So what are you waiting for?

CPSIA information can be obtained
at www.ICGtesting.com
Printed in the USA
LVHW080410220720
661015LV00024B/870

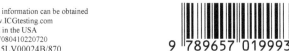